LOW FODMAP VEGETARIAN COOKBOOK

Nourishing Vegetarian Dishes for Digestive Wellness

Alex Kava

Copyright

Table of contents

Introduction

In a world where dietary trends come and go, the focus on digestive wellness remains steadfast as a cornerstone of overall health. The connection between what we eat and how our bodies function is undeniable, especially when it comes to our digestive system. Welcome to "Nourishing Vegetarian Dishes for Digestive Wellness," a culinary journey that marries the principles of the Low FODMAP diet with the delicious creativity of vegetarian cuisine.

Understanding the Low FODMAP Diet

The Low FODMAP diet has gained recognition for its efficacy in managing irritable bowel syndrome (IBS) and other gastrointestinal issues. FODMAPs, short for Fermentable Oligosaccharides, Disaccharides, Monosaccharides, and Polyols, are a group of carbohydrates that can trigger digestive discomfort in susceptible individuals. By avoiding high FODMAP foods, many people have found relief from bloating, gas, abdominal pain, and irregular bowel movements.

This cookbook is a celebration of the symbiosis between a vegetarian lifestyle and the Low FODMAP approach. While the Low FODMAP diet can be restrictive, especially for vegetarians, our aim is to showcase that nourishing, flavorful, and satisfying meals are not only possible but abundant within these dietary guidelines.

Benefits of a Vegetarian Approach

Embracing a vegetarian lifestyle brings its own set of health benefits, ranging from reduced risk of chronic diseases to positive impacts on the environment. A well-balanced vegetarian diet is rich in plant-based foods like vegetables, fruits, legumes, nuts, and seeds. These foods are packed with essential nutrients, antioxidants, and dietary fiber that support digestive health, provide sustained energy, and contribute to overall vitality.

This cookbook strives to bridge the gap between the Low FODMAP and vegetarian lifestyles, empowering you to embark on a journey that supports both your digestive wellness and your ethical dietary choices.

Tips for Digestive Wellness

Before we embark on this flavorful journey, let's explore some fundamental tips for maintaining digestive wellness:

1. Mindful Eating: Take time to savor and chew your food. Eating slowly aids digestion and allows you to recognize when you're full.

2. Hydration: Drink an adequate amount of water throughout the day to keep your digestive system functioning optimally.

3. Fiber-Rich Foods: Incorporate a variety of fiber-rich foods to support regular bowel movements and nourish your gut microbiome.

4. Probiotic Foods: Include fermented foods like yogurt, kefir, and sauerkraut to promote a healthy balance of gut bacteria.

5. Stress Management: Practicing stress-reduction techniques, such as meditation, yoga, or deep breathing, can positively impact your digestive system.

6. Balanced Meals: Aim for balanced meals that include a combination of protein, healthy fats, and complex carbohydrates to stabilize blood sugar levels and aid digestion.

7. Portion Control: Pay attention to portion sizes to prevent overeating, which can strain your digestive system.

In the pages that follow, you'll discover a treasure trove of plant-based recipes meticulously crafted to be both delicious and supportive of your digestive well-being. From hearty breakfasts to satisfying dinners, flavorful snacks to delectable desserts, our goal is to provide you with a diverse array of options that align with the Low FODMAP and vegetarian principles.

So, let's embark on this flavorful journey together, as we explore the world of Nourishing Vegetarian Dishes for Digestive Wellness. May your culinary endeavors not only tantalize your taste buds but also nurture your body and soul.

Chapter 1: Understanding the Low FODMAP Diet

In the quest for optimal digestive wellness, the Low FODMAP diet has emerged as a valuable tool, offering relief to those grappling with irritable bowel syndrome (IBS) and other gastrointestinal sensitivities. FODMAPs, a complex group of fermentable carbohydrates, have garnered attention for their potential to trigger discomfort in susceptible individuals. Let's delve into the intricacies of the Low FODMAP diet, shedding light on its principles and its role in promoting digestive harmony.

Unveiling FODMAPs: Fermentable Carbohydrates and Digestive Distress

FODMAPs, an acronym that stands for Fermentable Oligosaccharides, Disaccharides, Monosaccharides, and Polyols, encompass a diverse range of carbohydrates found in various foods. For individuals with sensitive digestive systems, consuming high FODMAP foods can lead to a cascade of uncomfortable symptoms, including bloating, gas, abdominal pain, diarrhea, and constipation.

1. Oligosaccharides: These include fructans and galacto-oligosaccharides (GOS), found in foods like wheat, onions, garlic, and legumes.

2. Disaccharides: Lactose, a disaccharide present in dairy products, can pose challenges for those with lactose intolerance.

3. Monosaccharides: Fructose, found in honey, certain fruits, and high fructose corn syrup, can be problematic when consumed in excess of glucose.

4. Polyols: Sugar alcohols such as sorbitol, mannitol, xylitol, and maltitol are commonly added to sugar-free products and occur naturally in some fruits and vegetables.

The Low FODMAP Approach: Easing Digestive Discomfort

The Low FODMAP diet is rooted in the principle of reducing the consumption of high FODMAP foods, thereby alleviating gastrointestinal symptoms. This dietary strategy involves a structured elimination phase followed by a reintroduction phase to identify specific trigger foods for each individual.

Elimination Phase: During this phase, high FODMAP foods are temporarily removed from the diet. This allows the gut to rest and symptoms to subside, providing a clearer baseline for assessing food sensitivities.

Reintroduction Phase: Gradually, FODMAP-containing foods are reintroduced in controlled portions to pinpoint which ones trigger symptoms. This personalized approach empowers individuals to create a tailored, sustainable eating plan.

Ongoing Maintenance: Once trigger foods are identified, a modified diet is developed to suit an individual's digestive needs while maximizing nutritional intake.

Low FODMAP and Vegetarian Harmony

For vegetarians, the Low FODMAP diet might seem challenging due to the prominence of high FODMAP foods in plant-based sources such as legumes, onions, and certain fruits. However, this cookbook seeks to bridge the gap by offering a wide array of flavorful, nourishing vegetarian recipes that adhere to the principles of both dietary lifestyles.

By focusing on low FODMAP vegetables, grains, nuts, seeds, and other plant-based ingredients, we've crafted recipes that allow vegetarians to savor the benefits of this diet without sacrificing taste or nutrition. The pages that follow are a testament to the harmonious blend of digestive sensitivity and ethical dietary choices.

As we embark on this culinary journey, remember that understanding the Low FODMAP diet is the first step toward fostering a healthier relationship with your digestive system. With knowledge as our guide, we are better equipped to make informed choices that pave the way for enhanced well-being and renewed vitality. So, let's turn the page and explore the world of nourishing vegetarian dishes designed to support digestive wellness in every mouthwatering bite.

Benefits of a Vegetarian Approach

In a world where dietary choices have profound implications for our health and the environment, embracing a vegetarian lifestyle has garnered widespread recognition for its multifaceted benefits. As we embark on a journey of digestive wellness through the lens of the Low FODMAP diet, it becomes evident that a vegetarian approach not only aligns harmoniously but also amplifies the positive impact on our well-being. Let's delve into the abundant advantages that a vegetarian diet brings to the table.

Nourishing with Plant-Powered Nutrients

A well-planned vegetarian diet centers around whole, plant-based foods rich in essential nutrients that contribute to optimal digestive function and overall health. By prioritizing a diverse range of vegetables, fruits, legumes, nuts, seeds, and whole grains, vegetarians effortlessly access an array of vitamins, minerals, antioxidants, and dietary fiber. These components are instrumental in supporting digestive health, regulating bowel movements, and fostering a balanced gut microbiome.

Digestive Harmony Through Dietary Fiber

Dietary fiber is a cornerstone of digestive wellness, and vegetarian diets are naturally abundant in this essential nutrient. Fiber adds bulk to stools, aiding in regular bowel movements and preventing constipation. Moreover, certain soluble fibers found in foods like oats, legumes, and fruits can help regulate blood sugar levels and promote satiety, contributing to a stable digestive rhythm.

Reducing Gastrointestinal Stress

Vegetarian diets often incorporate less processed and fatty foods compared to omnivorous diets. This can lead to reduced stress on the digestive system, allowing it to operate more efficiently. The absence of red meat, which can be harder to digest for some individuals, can alleviate digestive strain and contribute to a lighter, more comfortable feeling after meals.

Promoting Gut Microbiome Diversity

A flourishing gut microbiome is pivotal to digestive health and overall well-being. Vegetarian diets, rich in plant-based fibers, prebiotics, and polyphenols, provide an optimal environment for a diverse and thriving community of gut bacteria. A balanced gut microbiome is associated with improved digestion, enhanced nutrient absorption, and reduced inflammation – all essential components of digestive wellness.

Eco-Friendly and Ethical Considerations

Beyond personal health, choosing a vegetarian diet aligns with environmentally conscious and ethical values. Animal agriculture is a significant contributor to greenhouse gas emissions and environmental degradation. By embracing plant-based eating, you contribute to reducing your carbon footprint and promoting sustainable food practices that benefit both the planet and future generations.

Cultivating Mindful Eating Habits

Vegetarianism encourages a deeper connection to food and a heightened awareness of what we consume. This mindful approach to eating can translate to improved digestion, as it fosters slower and more conscious eating habits. Chewing thoroughly and savoring each bite allows the body to better process and absorb nutrients, promoting digestive efficiency.

As we embark on this journey of crafting nourishing vegetarian dishes tailored to the principles of the

Low FODMAP diet, let's celebrate the harmonious interplay between a plant-based lifestyle and digestive wellness. In the pages that follow, you'll discover a plethora of culinary creations that not only delight the palate but also empower you to experience the transformative benefits of embracing a vegetarian approach to nourishment. So, let's dive into this tapestry of flavors and nutrients, as we cultivate a deep sense of well-being that resonates from within.

Tips for Digestive Wellness

In the intricate dance of health and vitality, our digestive system takes center stage as a conductor orchestrating the harmonious rhythm of our well-being. Nurturing this complex symphony requires a symphony of care, attention, and mindful choices. As we embark on a journey to explore nourishing vegetarian dishes that embrace the principles of the Low FODMAP diet, it's essential to equip ourselves with a treasure trove of tips and techniques that will guide us toward digestive wellness.

Honoring Your Digestive Temple

Imagine your digestive system as a temple – a sacred space where the alchemy of digestion occurs. The foods we choose to nourish this temple have a profound impact on our overall health and vitality. To honor this intricate process, we must approach our dietary choices with reverence and mindfulness.

The Art of Mindful Eating

Mindful eating is a practice that invites us to engage all our senses in the act of nourishment. It encourages us to savor each bite, appreciate the flavors and textures, and be present in the moment. By slowing down and paying attention to our meals, we allow our bodies to fully process and absorb nutrients, supporting optimal digestion.

Hydration and Digestive Vigor

Just as a river flows smoothly, our digestive system thrives when it's well-hydrated. Drinking an ample amount of water throughout the day ensures that the digestive process is well-lubricated, facilitating the movement of food through the gastrointestinal tract. Hydration also helps prevent constipation and supports the body in breaking down and absorbing nutrients.

The Power of Dietary Fiber

Dietary fiber acts as a broom, gently sweeping away waste and toxins from our digestive tract. A diet rich in fiber from fruits, vegetables, whole grains, legumes, and seeds helps regulate bowel movements and promotes a feeling of fullness. Fiber also serves as a prebiotic, nourishing the beneficial bacteria in our gut and contributing to a balanced microbiome.

Balanced and Wholesome Meals

Crafting meals that strike a harmonious balance between protein, healthy fats, and complex carbohydrates is key to supporting digestion. Balanced meals provide sustained energy, prevent blood sugar spikes, and facilitate the breakdown and absorption of nutrients. Incorporating a variety of colorful vegetables further enhances the nutrient profile of your meals.

Stress Reduction for Digestive Ease

The mind and the gut are intimately connected, and stress can manifest physically in the form of digestive discomfort. Engaging in stress-reducing practices such as meditation, deep breathing, yoga, and mindfulness can have a profound impact on digestive wellness. By calming the mind, we create an environment conducive to optimal digestion.

Portion Awareness and Mindful Satiety

Understanding portion sizes and recognizing satiety cues are essential for promoting comfortable digestion. Overeating can strain the digestive system, leading to discomfort and sluggishness. Listening to your body and eating until you feel satisfied, rather than overly full, allows for a smoother digestive process.

As we embark on this exploration of tips for digestive wellness, remember that these practices are not isolated steps but interconnected threads in the tapestry of health. By cultivating mindfulness, making conscious dietary choices, and embracing practices that support our unique digestive systems, we set the stage for a symphony of well-being that resonates within us. In the chapters that follow, we will dive deeper into the world of nourishing vegetarian dishes crafted to honor our digestive temples and nurture our overall vitality. So, let's journey onward with an open heart and a nourished spirit, ready to embrace the transformative power of mindful digestion.

Chapter 2: Getting Started with the Low FODMAP Vegetarian Lifestyle

Embarking on the path of the Low FODMAP vegetarian lifestyle is an exciting and empowering journey toward enhanced digestive wellness. This section serves as your compass, guiding you through the foundational principles and practical steps to seamlessly integrate this approach into your daily life. Whether you're a long-time vegetarian looking to refine your dietary choices or a newcomer seeking digestive relief, this chapter equips you with the knowledge and tools to navigate this rewarding path.

The Basics of Low FODMAP Eating

At the heart of the Low FODMAP diet lies a commitment to reducing the consumption of specific types of fermentable carbohydrates that can trigger digestive discomfort. As you transition to a Low FODMAP vegetarian lifestyle, it's important to familiarize yourself with the categories of FODMAPs – Fermentable Oligosaccharides, Disaccharides, Monosaccharides, and Polyols – and the foods that fall within each category.

Vegetarian Sources of Essential Nutrients

Adopting a vegetarian lifestyle while following the Low FODMAP diet requires thoughtful consideration of nutrient intake. While some high FODMAP plant-based foods are restricted, a world of nutrient-rich options remains at your disposal. Discover alternative sources of essential nutrients such as protein, iron, calcium, vitamin B12, omega-3 fatty acids, and zinc within the framework of Low FODMAP vegetarian eating.

Meal Planning and Grocery Shopping

Efficient meal planning and strategic grocery shopping are key components of a successful Low

FODMAP vegetarian lifestyle. Learn how to curate a well-balanced, nourishing menu that aligns with your dietary goals. Armed with a list of Low FODMAP vegetarian staples and a selection of vibrant fruits, vegetables, whole grains, legumes, nuts, and seeds, you'll be ready to create culinary masterpieces that support your digestive wellness.

Navigating Recipe Modifications and Substitutions

Adapting traditional recipes to suit the Low FODMAP vegetarian lifestyle requires creativity and a willingness to explore new flavors and ingredients. Uncover the art of recipe modifications and substitutions that retain the essence of your favorite dishes while adhering to the principles of this dietary approach. Discover low FODMAP swaps for onions, garlic, and other high FODMAP ingredients, ensuring that each bite is both flavorful and gentle on your digestion.

Cultivating Mindful Eating Habits

Mindful eating is a cornerstone of the Low FODMAP vegetarian lifestyle, nurturing a deeper connection between your body and the food you consume. Explore techniques for practicing mindful eating, including savoring each bite, recognizing hunger and fullness cues, and fostering a present-centered relationship with your meals. By embracing mindfulness, you enhance the digestion of nutrients and heighten your overall dining experience.

As you embark on your journey into the world of Low FODMAP vegetarian living, remember that each step you take toward enhanced digestive wellness is an investment in your long-term health and vitality. With a foundation of knowledge, a pantry stocked with nourishing ingredients, and a willingness to explore new culinary horizons, you're well-prepared to craft a dietary landscape that supports both your digestive needs and your ethical choices. Let's venture forward, embracing the joys of Low FODMAP vegetarian cooking and celebrating the symphony of flavors and well-being that it brings.

The Basics of Low FODMAP Eating

Embarking on a Low FODMAP vegetarian lifestyle is a transformative step toward nurturing your digestive wellness while embracing a plant-based diet. To embark on this journey with confidence and clarity, it's essential to grasp the fundamental principles of Low FODMAP eating. In this section, we delve into the intricacies of FODMAPs and guide you through the process of identifying and enjoying Low FODMAP foods as a vegetarian.

Unveiling the World of FODMAPs

FODMAPs, an acronym for Fermentable Oligosaccharides, Disaccharides, Monosaccharides, and Polyols, represent a group of carbohydrates that can trigger digestive discomfort in susceptible individuals. Understanding each category is pivotal to navigating the Low FODMAP vegetarian lifestyle:

1. **Oligosaccharides:** These include fructans (found in wheat, onions, garlic) and galacto-oligosaccharides (found in legumes).

2. **Disaccharides:** Lactose, present in dairy products, can be challenging for some individuals to digest.

3. **Monosaccharides:** Fructose (found in certain fruits, honey) can pose problems when consumed in excess of glucose.

4. **Polyols:** Sugar alcohols like sorbitol, mannitol, and xylitol are found naturally in some fruits and are commonly used as sweeteners.

The Low FODMAP Approach

The Low FODMAP approach involves reducing high FODMAP foods from your diet to alleviate digestive discomfort and promote wellness. For vegetarians, this may involve adjustments to traditional dietary choices while embracing a rich tapestry of low FODMAP plant-based foods.

Remember that not all high FODMAP foods need to be entirely eliminated; portion sizes and combinations play a role in maintaining digestive harmony.

Navigating High and Low FODMAP Foods as a Vegetarian

Vegetarian staples like legumes, wheat-based products, and certain fruits and vegetables can be high in FODMAPs. However, a wealth of Low FODMAP alternatives exists within the vegetarian realm. Opt for low FODMAP vegetables such as carrots, bell peppers, and spinach. Enjoy grains like quinoa, rice, and oats in moderation. Experiment with tofu, tempeh, and plant-based protein sources that align with the Low FODMAP diet.

Building Balanced Meals

Creating balanced meals is paramount in the Low FODMAP vegetarian lifestyle. Strive for a harmonious combination of Low FODMAP protein sources, grains, and a colorful array of vegetables.

This not only supports your digestive system but also ensures a comprehensive intake of essential nutrients.

Mindful Meal Preparation and Portion Control

Approach meal preparation mindfully, incorporating cooking techniques that enhance digestibility. Steaming, roasting, and grilling can bring out flavors without compromising FODMAP content. Additionally, practice portion control to prevent overloading your digestive system and to promote comfortable eating experiences.

As you embark on your journey into the world of Low FODMAP vegetarian eating, remember that knowledge is your ally. The foundation you build in understanding FODMAPs and making informed food choices will empower you to create meals that nurture both your digestive wellness and your vegetarian values. In the chapters that follow, you'll uncover a multitude of delightful, low FODMAP vegetarian recipes that invite you to savor every bite while honoring your body's unique needs. Let's journey onward, nourishing ourselves from within and embracing the joys of a vibrant and harmonious dietary lifestyle.

Vegetarian Sources of Essential Nutrients

Embracing a Low FODMAP vegetarian lifestyle is not just about adhering to dietary restrictions; it's an opportunity to celebrate the diverse and nutrient-rich world of plant-based foods. As a vegetarian, you can harness the power of Low FODMAP ingredients to create meals that not only support your digestive wellness but also provide a robust array of essential nutrients. In this section, we explore the key nutrients that are vital for your well-being and how you can source them within the framework of the Low FODMAP diet.

Plant-Powered Protein

Protein is an essential building block for maintaining and repairing tissues in your body.

While some high FODMAP vegetarian protein sources like beans and lentils may be limited, you still have plenty of options. Consider incorporating:

- **Tofu:** A versatile soy-based protein that can be grilled, stir-fried, or added to soups.
- **Tempeh:** A fermented soy product with a nutty flavor, rich in protein and probiotics.
- **Quinoa:** A complete protein source that can be used as a base for salads, bowls, and more.
- **Nuts and Seeds:** Almonds, walnuts, chia seeds, and pumpkin seeds provide both protein and healthy fats.

Iron-Rich Foods

Iron is crucial for oxygen transport and energy production. While certain high FODMAP plant-based iron sources like lentils and beans might be limited, you can turn to Low FODMAP alternatives such as:

- **Spinach:** A versatile leafy green that can be used in salads, smoothies, and cooked dishes.

- **Pumpkin Seeds:** These seeds offer a good dose of iron and can be sprinkled on various dishes.
- **Quinoa:** Apart from protein, quinoa is also a source of iron.
- **Tofu and Tempeh:** These soy-based products provide iron while also being protein-rich.

Calcium Considerations

Calcium is essential for strong bones and teeth. While dairy products are often a primary source of calcium, as a vegetarian, you have alternatives that fit the Low FODMAP profile:

- **Lactose-Free Dairy:** Lactose-free milk, cheese, and yogurt are suitable options.
- **Fortified Plant-Based Milks:** Almond, rice, and coconut milks fortified with calcium can be used as dairy alternatives.
- **Leafy Greens:** Kale, bok choy, and collard greens are Low FODMAP sources of calcium.
- **Canned Fish with Bones:** Certain canned fish like salmon and sardines contain edible bones and are high in calcium.

Vitamin B12 and Omega-3 Fatty Acids

Vitamin B12 is primarily found in animal products, making it essential for vegetarians to ensure adequate intake. Consider:

- **Fortified Foods:** Breakfast cereals, plant-based milks, and nutritional yeast often contain added vitamin B12.
- **Eggs:** If your vegetarian diet includes eggs, they can be a source of vitamin B12.
- **Omega-3-Rich Foods:** Flaxseeds and walnuts provide omega-3 fatty acids, essential for heart and brain health.

Zinc-Rich Vegetarian Options

Zinc is crucial for immune function, wound healing, and maintaining a healthy sense of taste and smell. Seek out:

- **Pumpkin Seeds:** Besides iron, pumpkin seeds are also a good source of zinc.

- **Tofu and Tempeh:** These soy-based options offer both protein and zinc.
- **Fortified Foods:** Some fortified plant-based foods may also provide zinc.

As you embark on your Low FODMAP vegetarian journey, remember that while certain nutrient-rich plant-based foods are limited due to FODMAP restrictions, there's a world of alternatives that can nourish you and support your well-being. By thoughtfully selecting a variety of Low FODMAP foods rich in essential nutrients, you're building a foundation for digestive wellness that resonates through every meal you create. In the next chapter, we'll explore the art of meal planning and grocery shopping to help you stock your kitchen with ingredients that align with your dietary goals and nutritional needs.

Meal Planning and Grocery Shopping

Embracing a low FODMAP (Fermentable Oligosaccharides, Disaccharides, Monosaccharides, and Polyols) vegetarian lifestyle can be an effective way to manage digestive issues such as irritable bowel syndrome (IBS). The low FODMAP diet involves avoiding specific types of carbohydrates that are poorly absorbed by the small intestine, which can trigger symptoms like bloating, gas, and abdominal pain. For those choosing to follow a vegetarian path within the framework of this diet, careful meal planning and strategic grocery shopping are essential to ensure a well-balanced and satisfying diet. This guide will provide you with practical insights on how to get started with the low FODMAP vegetarian lifestyle, focusing on meal planning and grocery shopping strategies.

1. Understand the Low FODMAP Vegetarian Diet:

Before embarking on this dietary journey, it's important to familiarize yourself with both the low FODMAP and vegetarian diets. Learn about the types of foods that are high and low in FODMAPs, as well as vegetarian sources of essential nutrients like protein, iron, calcium, and vitamin B12. Seek guidance from a registered dietitian to ensure you're meeting your nutritional needs.

2. Create a List of Low FODMAP Vegetables, Fruits, Grains, and Legumes:

Compile a list of low FODMAP vegetarian foods that you can include in your meals. Some examples include carrots, bell peppers, spinach, zucchini, strawberries, blueberries, quinoa, rice, oats, and lentils. Having this list handy will simplify the process of meal planning and grocery shopping.

3. Plan Balanced Meals:

Aim for balanced meals that incorporate a variety of nutrient-rich foods. Combine low FODMAP vegetables, fruits, grains, and legumes to create satisfying and nourishing dishes. Prioritize sources of plant-based protein like tofu, tempeh, eggs, and lactose-free dairy products.

4. Experiment with Recipes:

Explore low FODMAP vegetarian recipes to add diversity to your diet. Experiment with different cooking methods and seasonings to enhance flavors without triggering digestive discomfort. Incorporate herbs, spices, and low FODMAP condiments to elevate your meals.

5. Incorporate Adequate Fiber:

Since some high-fiber foods can be high in FODMAPs, it's important to find sources of soluble and insoluble fiber that are safe for your diet. Chia seeds, flaxseeds, and psyllium husk are low FODMAP options that can help maintain healthy digestion.

6. Plan Ahead:

Set aside time each week to plan your meals and snacks. Create a weekly meal schedule that includes a variety of dishes. This will not only save you time during busy weekdays but also ensure that you have balanced and satisfying options readily available.

7. Make a Shopping List:

Based on your meal plan, create a detailed shopping list. Include specific quantities of ingredients to avoid food waste. Prioritize fresh produce, lean proteins, and pantry staples. Check your list against your list of low FODMAP foods to ensure that you're purchasing suitable options.

8. Read Labels Carefully:

When shopping for packaged foods, carefully read labels to identify any high FODMAP ingredients. Look out for hidden sources of FODMAPs, such as onion and garlic powders, high fructose corn syrup, and certain artificial sweeteners.

9. Explore FODMAP-Friendly Substitutes:

Some high FODMAP ingredients can be substituted with low FODMAP alternatives. For instance, use garlic-infused oil instead of whole garlic cloves for flavor, or opt for lactose-free dairy products to meet your calcium needs.

10. Be Mindful of Portion Sizes:

Even low FODMAP foods can trigger symptoms if consumed in excessive amounts. Pay attention to portion sizes and listen to your body's signals. Gradually introduce new foods to gauge your tolerance.

Embracing a low FODMAP vegetarian lifestyle requires thoughtful meal planning and strategic grocery shopping. By understanding the principles of the low FODMAP diet and selecting a variety of nutrient-rich vegetarian foods, you can create satisfying and well-balanced meals that support your digestive health. With careful planning, experimentation, and attention to your body's responses, you can navigate this dietary journey successfully and enjoy the benefits of improved well-being. Remember to consult a healthcare professional or registered dietitian before making significant changes to your diet, especially if you have underlying health conditions.

Chapter 3: Breakfasts to Fuel Your Day

They say that breakfast is the most important meal of the day, and for good reason. A well-balanced breakfast provides your body with the essential nutrients and energy it needs to kickstart your day on the right foot. Whether you have a busy schedule ahead or a leisurely morning to enjoy, choosing the right breakfast can set the tone for your entire day. Here are some delicious and nutritious breakfast options that will help fuel your day and keep you going strong:

1. Classic Oatmeal Power Bowl: Start your morning with a classic bowl of oatmeal. Oats are rich in fiber, which helps maintain steady blood sugar levels and keeps you feeling full. Top your oatmeal with a variety of toppings such as fresh berries, sliced bananas, chopped nuts, and a drizzle of honey or maple syrup for a touch of natural sweetness.

2. Protein-Packed Smoothie: Blend up a smoothie that's not only delicious but also packed with protein. Combine your favorite protein powder with almond milk, a handful of spinach or kale, a scoop of nut butter, and some frozen fruits like berries or mango. This nutrient-packed concoction will provide you with a quick and convenient burst of energy.

3. Avocado Toast with Eggs: Avocado toast has become a breakfast staple for a reason. Spread ripe avocado on whole-grain toast and top it with poached or scrambled eggs. Avocado offers healthy fats while eggs provide protein, creating a balanced and satisfying meal.

4. Greek Yogurt Parfait: Greek yogurt is a fantastic source of protein and probiotics. Layer it with granola, mixed berries, and a drizzle of honey for a parfait that not only pleases your taste buds but also supports your digestive health.

5. Veggie-Packed Breakfast Burrito: Wrap scrambled eggs, sautéed veggies, and a sprinkle of cheese in a whole-wheat tortilla to create a hearty breakfast burrito. The combination of protein, fiber, and vitamins from the vegetables will keep you fueled for hours.

6. Homemade Energy Bars: If you're on the go, whip up a batch of homemade energy bars using oats, nuts, dried fruits, and a touch of honey or dates for natural sweetness. These bars are a convenient and nutritious option for those rushed mornings.

7. Quinoa Breakfast Bowl: Swap out your usual grains for quinoa, a complete protein source. Cook quinoa and top it with sliced almonds, chopped fruits like apples or pears, and a sprinkle of cinnamon for a warm and satisfying breakfast.

8. Whole-Grain Pancakes/Waffles: Indulge in whole-grain pancakes or waffles topped with fresh fruit and a dollop of Greek yogurt. Opt for whole-grain varieties to increase fiber content and pair them with your favorite nutritious toppings.

9. Chia Seed Pudding: Prepare chia seed pudding the night before by mixing chia seeds with your choice of milk and a touch of vanilla extract. Let it sit in the fridge overnight to thicken. In the morning, top it with fruits, nuts, and a drizzle of agave syrup.

10. Smoked Salmon Toast: For a savory option, top whole-grain toast with cream cheese, smoked salmon, capers, and red onion slices. This combination provides omega-3 fatty acids, protein, and a burst of flavors to awaken your taste buds.

The key to a breakfast that truly fuels your day is a balance of protein, healthy fats, and complex carbohydrates. By choosing nutrient-dense ingredients and experimenting with different combinations, you can create breakfasts that not only satisfy your hunger but also provide the energy you need to conquer whatever comes your way. So, rise and shine with these nourishing breakfast ideas and make the most out of your mornings!

Quinoa and Blueberry Breakfast Bowl

In the world of breakfast options, the Quinoa and Blueberry Breakfast Bowl stands out as a nutritional powerhouse that can kickstart your day with energy and vitality. This delightful bowl brings together the goodness of quinoa, the sweetness of blueberries, and a variety of complementary ingredients to create a delicious and nutritious morning meal.

The Quinoa Base:

Quinoa, often referred to as a superfood, is a complete protein source packed with essential amino acids. It's also a rich source of dietary fiber, providing a slow release of energy to keep you feeling full and focused throughout the morning. Begin your breakfast by cooking quinoa according to the package instructions. Fluff it with a fork and set it as the hearty base of your bowl.

Blueberry Bliss:

Blueberries, known for their vibrant color and antioxidant content, add a burst of flavor and health benefits to your breakfast. These little berries are packed with vitamins, minerals, and powerful antioxidants that support brain health, boost your immune system, and contribute to healthy skin. Add a generous handful of fresh blueberries to your quinoa base.

Creamy Greek Yogurt:

Greek yogurt is a creamy and protein-rich addition that complements the nutty texture of quinoa and the juicy burst of blueberries. It's a probiotic powerhouse that supports gut health and provides a satisfying creaminess to your breakfast bowl. Dollop a generous spoonful of Greek yogurt on top of your blueberries.

Crunchy Nutty Toppings:

For an added layer of texture and flavor, sprinkle your breakfast bowl with a mix of chopped nuts and seeds. Almonds, walnuts, and chia seeds are excellent choices. These ingredients not only contribute healthy fats but also provide a satisfying crunch that contrasts with the creamy yogurt and tender quinoa.

Drizzle of Honey or Maple Syrup:

To enhance the natural sweetness of the blueberries and yogurt, consider drizzling a touch of honey or maple syrup over the top of your bowl. These natural sweeteners add a touch of indulgence while providing a quick source of energy.

Optional Additions:

Feel free to customize your Quinoa and Blueberry Breakfast Bowl to your taste preferences and nutritional needs. Sliced bananas, diced apples, or even a sprinkle of cinnamon can take this breakfast to the next level. If you're looking to boost your protein intake, consider adding a scoop of your favorite protein powder to the yogurt or incorporating a handful of chopped hard-boiled eggs.

With its blend of protein, fiber, antioxidants, and healthy fats, the Quinoa and Blueberry Breakfast Bowl offers a balanced and satisfying way to fuel your day. This breakfast not only provides sustained energy but also supports your overall well-being, making it a fantastic choice for those who want to start their mornings on a nutritious note.

Overnight Chia Seed Pudding

Looking for a breakfast that's not only convenient but also incredibly nutritious? Overnight Chia Seed Pudding might just be your new morning favorite. This delightful dish offers a perfect balance of flavors and textures while providing a hearty dose of essential nutrients to kickstart your day.

The Chia Seed Base:
Chia seeds are small but mighty powerhouses of nutrition. They are rich in fiber, protein, and healthy fats, making them an excellent choice to keep you feeling full and satisfied. When soaked in liquid, chia seeds form a gel-like consistency that resembles pudding. To create your base, mix chia seeds with your choice of milk (dairy or plant-

based) in a jar or bowl. The general ratio is about 1/4 cup of chia seeds to 1 cup of liquid.

Creamy and Customizable:

One of the beauties of overnight chia seed pudding is its versatility. You can customize it to suit your taste preferences. For a creamy and indulgent pudding, opt for coconut milk or almond milk. If you prefer a lighter option, go for skim milk or a nut-free milk alternative. Add a touch of vanilla extract and a drizzle of honey or maple syrup to enhance the flavor.

Flavor Infusion:

While the chia seeds work their magic overnight, you can infuse your pudding with a variety of flavors. Mix in a tablespoon of cocoa powder for a chocolate twist, or stir in a teaspoon of matcha powder for a vibrant and energizing green hue. Alternatively, you can add a sprinkle of cinnamon, nutmeg, or even a dash of cardamom for a warm and comforting flavor profile.

Top it Off:

In the morning, your chia seed pudding will have transformed into a velvety and satisfying texture. Now, it's time to get creative with your toppings. Fresh fruits like berries, sliced bananas, or diced mangoes add a burst of natural sweetness and a dose of vitamins. Chopped nuts, toasted coconut flakes, and granola provide a delightful crunch and additional nutritional value.

The Nutrient Boost:

Aside from being a great source of fiber and healthy fats, chia seeds are loaded with omega-3 fatty acids, antioxidants, and various vitamins and minerals. These tiny seeds offer benefits such as improved digestion, heart health, and stable blood sugar levels. By starting your day with a chia seed pudding, you're nourishing your body with essential nutrients that support your overall well-being.

Preparation Made Easy:

One of the most appealing aspects of overnight chia seed pudding is its simplicity. You can prepare it the night before, allowing the chia seeds to absorb the liquid and create that pudding-like texture while you sleep. In the morning, your breakfast is ready to enjoy without any fuss or cooking required.

Overnight Chia Seed Pudding is not only a convenient breakfast option but also a delicious and nutrient-dense way to fuel your day. With its endless possibilities for customization and its impressive health benefits, this breakfast dish is a perfect addition to your morning routine. So, embrace the magic of chia seeds and start your day with a bowl of creamy, satisfying, and energizing goodness.

Zucchini and Carrot Muffins

When it comes to breakfast, the Zucchini and Carrot Muffins offer a delightful twist that combines wholesome ingredients with undeniable flavor. These muffins are not only a tasty treat but also a nutritious way to kickstart your morning and keep you energized throughout the day.

The Veggie Powerhouse:

Zucchini and carrots are the stars of this breakfast creation. Packed with vitamins, minerals, and dietary fiber, these vegetables provide a nutritional boost to your muffins. The addition of zucchini and carrots adds moisture, texture, and a hint of natural sweetness, making these muffins both delectable and nourishing.

Whole Grain Goodness:

To ensure that your breakfast is rich in complex carbohydrates and dietary fiber, opt for whole grain flour as the base for your muffins. Whole grains release energy slowly, helping you maintain stable blood sugar levels and feel full for longer periods. Whole wheat flour, oat flour, or a combination of flours can be used to create a hearty and satisfying muffin base.

Nutrient-Packed Add-Ins:

Enhance the nutritional content of your Zucchini and Carrot Muffins by incorporating nutrient-rich ingredients. Chopped nuts like walnuts or almonds provide healthy fats and crunch, while dried fruits like raisins or cranberries add natural sweetness and a burst of flavor. You can also consider mixing in a handful of seeds such as sunflower seeds or chia seeds for added texture and health benefits.

Natural Sweeteners:

Keep your muffins on the healthier side by using natural sweeteners. A touch of honey, maple syrup, or mashed ripe banana can provide the right amount of sweetness without the need for refined sugars. These options not only add flavor but also offer additional nutrients and antioxidants.

Spices and Flavors:

To elevate the taste of your muffins, experiment with a variety of spices and flavors. Cinnamon, nutmeg, and ginger can add warmth and depth to the muffins, creating a cozy and inviting aroma as they bake. A splash of vanilla extract can enhance the overall flavor profile, making each bite a delightful experience.

Balanced and Satisfying:

The combination of vegetables, whole grains, and nutrient-dense add-ins ensures that your Zucchini and Carrot Muffins offer a balanced and satisfying breakfast option. The fiber from the vegetables and whole grains, along with the protein from nuts or seeds, provides a steady source of energy to fuel your day and keep you feeling satiated.

Make Ahead for Convenience:
Preparing a batch of Zucchini and Carrot Muffins in advance allows you to have a quick and convenient breakfast option throughout the week. Simply bake a batch during your free time, and store them in an airtight container. Grab a muffin on busy mornings or enjoy them as a mid-morning snack for a sustained energy boost.

By choosing Zucchini and Carrot Muffins as your breakfast of choice, you're treating yourself to a wholesome and flavorful start to the day. These muffins embody the perfect blend of nutrition and taste, making them a delightful addition to your breakfast repertoire. So, indulge in the goodness of vegetables and whole grains, and let these muffins fuel your day with vitality and satisfaction.

Chapter 4: Flavorful Soups and Satisfying Salads

In the world of gastronomy, few dishes manage to capture the essence of comfort and health quite like soups and salads. These two culinary powerhouses not only provide a burst of flavors and textures but also offer a nutritious and delightful dining experience. Whether enjoyed as a warm, hearty bowl on a chilly evening or a refreshing, crunchy plate on a scorching summer day, flavorful soups and satisfying salads have earned their place as versatile and beloved components of menus worldwide.

Savoring the Symphony of Soups:

Soups, with their steaming bowls of liquid goodness, have been cherished across cultures for centuries. From velvety purees to chunky broths, soups come in an array of forms, each offering a unique combination of flavors and aromas. Let's dive into the world of soups and explore their captivating qualities:

1. Broths and Bouillabaisse: These light yet deeply flavorful soups form the base of many culinary traditions. A simmering pot of bones, vegetables, herbs, and spices yields a nourishing broth that can be enjoyed on its own or serve as the foundation for heartier soups.

2. Creamy Elegance: Cream-based soups, like the classic tomato bisque or rich mushroom velouté, indulge the palate with their luxurious textures and velvety flavors. The interplay between creaminess and the subtle tang of ingredients makes these soups a favorite comfort food.

3. Hearty Stews: Stews blur the line between soup and main course, offering a wholesome amalgamation of vegetables, meats, and legumes. Whether it's a slow-cooked beef stew or a vibrant vegetarian chili, these one-pot wonders pack a punch of taste and comfort.

4. Exotic Infusions: Embark on a culinary adventure with exotic soups like pho from Vietnam, gazpacho from Spain, or laksa from Southeast Asia. These soups combine regional spices, herbs, and ingredients to create a symphony of flavors that transport your taste buds to distant lands.

Crafting Artful Salads:

On the flip side of the culinary spectrum, we have salads—vibrant, refreshing, and endlessly customizable. Salads have evolved far beyond mere greens and dressings; they've become a canvas for creative culinary expression. Let's explore the nuances of crafting satisfying salads:

1. Leafy Beginnings: A medley of crisp, fresh greens serves as the foundation of many salads. From delicate baby spinach to robust arugula, the choice of leaves sets the tone for the entire dish.

2. Protein Power: Adding protein transforms a salad into a substantial meal. Grilled chicken, seared tofu, succulent shrimp, or marinated steak not only provide sustenance but also introduce savory and textural dimensions.

3. Colorful Crunch: Incorporating an assortment of colorful vegetables adds visual appeal and a satisfying crunch. Vibrant bell peppers, juicy tomatoes, crunchy cucumbers, and earthy carrots contribute both flavor and texture to the salad.

4. Nuts, Seeds, and Cheeses: To elevate salads to a new level of taste and texture, ingredients like toasted nuts, seeds, and crumbled cheeses offer a delightful contrast. Whether it's the creaminess of goat cheese, the nuttiness of toasted almonds, or the subtle bite of sunflower seeds, these additions bring complexity to every bite.

5. Dress to Impress: The dressing is the finishing touch that ties all the components together. A well-balanced vinaigrette, creamy ranch, zesty citrus dressing, or tahini drizzle can enhance the flavors and ensure a harmonious flavor profile.

Harmony on the Plate:

In a world where culinary trends come and go, flavorful soups and satisfying salads remain steadfast fixtures on dining tables. They offer nourishment, comfort, and a playground for culinary creativity. Whether you're seeking warmth on a chilly day or a refreshing respite from the heat, these dishes deliver a symphony of flavors and textures that dance in harmony on the palate. So, the next time you savor a steaming bowl of soup or indulge in a vibrant salad, remember that you're not just enjoying a meal—you're experiencing a culinary journey that spans cultures, tastes, and time itself.

Roasted Red Pepper and Tomato Soup

In the realm of soups that embrace both comfort and culinary finesse, few options hold a candle to the captivating Roasted Red Pepper and Tomato Soup. This velvety concoction is a testament to the magic that unfolds when the simplicity of fresh ingredients combines with the artistry of preparation. A symphony of flavors awaits in every spoonful, making this soup a beloved classic that graces tables year-round.

The Elegance of Roasted Red Peppers and Tomatoes:

The foundation of this soup lies in the harmonious marriage of roasted red peppers and ripe tomatoes. The sweetness of the red peppers, transformed through the roasting process, plays a beautiful counterpoint to the natural acidity of tomatoes. When blended together, these ingredients create a base that's both lusciously smooth and intensely flavorful.

Crafting Culinary Alchemy:

Creating a Roasted Red Pepper and Tomato Soup is a journey that combines technique and intuition. Here's a glimpse into the process:

1. Roasting Brilliance: The red peppers take center stage as they are roasted until their skins blister and char, intensifying their inherent sweetness. This step infuses the soup with a smoky undertone that elevates the overall profile.

2. Tomato Tango: Ripe tomatoes, preferably of the plum variety, join the dance. These jewels of the garden contribute a vibrant acidity and depth of flavor that compliments the roasted peppers.

3. Aromatics and Harmony: Onions, garlic, and a medley of aromatic herbs and spices are sautéed to build a flavor foundation. The gentle sizzle releases their essential oils, infusing the kitchen with tantalizing aromas.

4. Blending Magic: The roasted red peppers, tomatoes, and sautéed aromatics come together in a blender, yielding a velvety mixture that's a feast for the eyes and the taste buds.

5. Creamy Indulgence: To achieve a luxurious texture, a touch of cream or a dairy-free alternative is introduced. This enriches the soup without overshadowing the starring ingredients, ensuring a harmonious balance.

6. Finishing Flourish: A final seasoning with salt, pepper, and perhaps a dash of paprika or cayenne pepper completes the symphony, accentuating the interplay of flavors.

A Feast for the Senses:

Serving Roasted Red Pepper and Tomato Soup is a sensory delight. The vibrant, fiery hue hints at the impending explosion of taste, while the aroma wafting from the bowl is enough to make mouths water. The first spoonful is a revelation—a harmonious blend of sweetness, acidity, and smokiness that dances on the palate.

Elevating the Experience with Sides:

To complement this flavorful soup, consider pairing it with a side salad that adds textural contrast and visual appeal. A simple mixed greens salad drizzled with a balsamic vinaigrette or a citrusy kale and quinoa salad can provide a satisfying crunch and balance to the richness of the soup.

Roasted Red Pepper and Tomato Soup is a timeless testament to the culinary art form's ability to transform humble ingredients into a masterpiece that warms the soul. This flavorful soup embodies the essence of both comfort and sophistication, making it an exceptional addition to any dining occasion. Whether enjoyed on a chilly evening or as a light indulgence during warmer months, this soup encapsulates the very essence of what makes flavorful soups and satisfying salads an integral part of the culinary landscape.

Mixed Greens with Roasted Tofu and Citrus Dressing

When it comes to crafting a truly satisfying salad, the marriage of fresh ingredients, contrasting textures, and a burst of vibrant flavors can transform a simple dish into a culinary masterpiece.

Enter the Mixed Greens with Roasted Tofu and Citrus Dressing—a delightful symphony of taste and nutrition that highlights the art of salad creation.

A Dance of Flavors and Textures:

This salad brings together an array of elements, each contributing to a harmonious and delightful experience:

1. Mixed Greens Medley: The star of the show is a mix of fresh and crisp greens. Tender baby spinach, peppery arugula, delicate butter lettuce, and robust kale intermingle to create a diverse base that forms the canvas for the salad's artistry.

2. Roasted Tofu Delight: Tofu, marinated and then roasted to perfection, adds a protein-rich element to the salad. The tofu's golden exterior gives way to a tender interior, providing a satisfying contrast to the greens.

3. Vibrant Citrus Infusion: The citrus dressing is where the magic truly unfolds. A blend of zesty oranges, tangy lemons, or limes, harmoniously combined with a drizzle of olive oil and a touch of honey or maple syrup, elevates the salad with a burst of refreshing and lively flavors.

4. Nutty Crunch: A sprinkle of toasted nuts—almonds, walnuts, or pistachios—adds a delightful crunch and nutty richness that complements the greens and tofu.

5. Cheese Elegance: A crumble of feta or goat cheese lends a creamy and slightly tangy element to the dish, providing depth and balance to the overall flavor profile.

Crafting Culinary Artistry:

Creating the Mixed Greens with Roasted Tofu and Citrus Dressing is a blend of preparation and creativity

1. Tofu Transformation: Tofu is marinated in a mixture of soy sauce, garlic, ginger, and a hint of sesame oil. This infuses the tofu with flavor before it's roasted until golden and slightly crispy.

2. Green Ensemble: A mixture of baby spinach, arugula, butter lettuce, and kale is washed, dried, and carefully combined to create a varied and visually appealing bed of greens.

3. Citrus Symphony: The citrus dressing is crafted by whisking together freshly squeezed citrus juices, olive oil, a touch of honey or maple syrup, and a pinch of salt and pepper. The result is a tangy, refreshing dressing that ties the elements of the salad together.

4. Artful Assembly: The marinated and roasted tofu is placed atop the bed of mixed greens. Toasted nuts and crumbled cheese are scattered over the ensemble, adding layers of texture and taste.

5. Dress to Impress: The citrus dressing is generously drizzled over the salad just before serving, infusing each bite with its invigorating and zesty essence.

A Wholesome Culinary Experience:

The Mixed Greens with Roasted Tofu and Citrus Dressing embodies the epitome of a satisfying and nourishing salad. With its array of flavors, textures, and visual appeal, this dish stands as a testament to the remarkable balance and creativity that can be achieved when crafting culinary artistry on a plate.

Whether enjoyed as a refreshing light meal on a warm day or as a vibrant accompaniment to a heartier dish, this salad embodies the very essence of what makes flavorful soups and satisfying salads an integral part of the culinary landscape—a celebration of taste, health, and the joy of eating well.

Chapter 5: Delightful Sides and Snacks

In the world of gastronomy, sides and snacks hold a special place. They are the unsung heroes of any meal, adding bursts of flavor, texture, and variety to the dining experience. While the main course often takes center stage, it's the delightful sides and snacks that can truly elevate a meal from ordinary to extraordinary. Whether you're hosting a gathering, enjoying a quiet evening at home, or looking to impress your taste buds, crafting delectable sides and snacks is an art that can be mastered with a little creativity and exploration.

The Art of Crafting Sides:

Sides, often referred to as accompaniments, play a crucial role in balancing a meal. They complement the main dish, providing contrast and depth to the overall flavor profile. From creamy mashed potatoes that melt in your mouth to vibrant roasted vegetables that offer a satisfying crunch, sides have the power to turn a simple meal into a memorable feast.

But why stop at the usual suspects? Experimentation is key when it comes to creating delightful sides. Think beyond the traditional and embrace global influences. How about tangy kimchi coleslaw or fragrant saffron-infused rice? Incorporating unexpected ingredients can lead to astonishingly delicious results.

The Charm of Snacking:

Snacking is an experience that transcends age and culture. Whether you're enjoying a movie night, taking a break at work, or entertaining guests, the right snacks can set the tone and enhance the moment. Sweet or savory, crunchy or creamy, snacks offer a quick indulgence that satisfies cravings and provides a mini culinary adventure.

The world of snacks has evolved far beyond a simple bag of chips or a handful of nuts. Today, gourmet popcorn with flavors ranging from truffle parmesan to sriracha-lime grace the shelves. Artisanal cheese platters paired with fruit preserves and nuts offer a sophisticated snacking experience. Even classic comfort foods like mini sliders, stuffed mushrooms, or bruschetta can be elevated to new heights with creative toppings and flavor combinations.

Creating Culinary Harmony:

The synergy between sides and snacks is where culinary magic truly happens. Picture a gathering where an array of Mediterranean-inspired mezze platters welcomes guests, inviting them to savor hummus, falafel, olives, and warm pita. Or imagine a cozy night in, complete with a charcuterie board adorned with an assortment of cheeses, crackers, dried fruits, and cured meats. The interplay between textures, tastes, and aromas creates a harmonious symphony of flavors that excites the palate and leaves a lasting impression.

In the realm of gastronomy, sides and snacks hold limitless potential for culinary exploration and delight. Whether you're aiming for a well-balanced meal or seeking an array of nibbles to please a crowd, the world of sides and snacks offers endless avenues for creativity and innovation. By embracing diverse ingredients, experimenting with cooking techniques, and crafting unexpected combinations, you can embark on a gastronomic journey that transforms ordinary moments into extraordinary experiences. So, why not embark on your own culinary adventure and discover the joy of delightful sides and snacks? Your taste buds will thank you.

Roasted Turmeric Cauliflower

In the realm of culinary exploration, few dishes can match the delightful fusion of flavors and textures found in roasted turmeric cauliflower. This golden-hued masterpiece takes humble cauliflower florets and transforms them into a mouthwatering side or snack that tantalizes the taste buds and offers a wealth of health benefits.

Unveiling the Magic of Turmeric:

At the heart of this delectable creation lies turmeric, a spice celebrated for its vibrant color and potent health properties. Curcumin, the active compound in turmeric, boasts anti-inflammatory and antioxidant qualities, making it a worthy addition to any diet. When paired with cauliflower and brought to life through roasting, turmeric infuses each floret with a warm and earthy essence, elevating both the flavor and the visual appeal.

Roasting: The Art of Transformation:

Roasting is a culinary technique that works wonders with cauliflower. As the florets are exposed to the gentle heat of the oven, they undergo a transformation that results in a perfect balance of tenderness and crispness. The natural sugars present in cauliflower caramelize, creating a delectable sweetness that harmonizes beautifully with the earthy tones of turmeric.

Crafting Roasted Turmeric Cauliflower:

Creating roasted turmeric cauliflower is a straightforward yet rewarding process. Begin by preheating your oven to a moderate temperature, usually around 400°F (200°C). While the oven heats, prepare the cauliflower by breaking it into bite-sized florets. In a mixing bowl, combine the cauliflower florets with a drizzle of olive oil, ensuring each piece is lightly coated. Now, the star of the show enters: turmeric. Sprinkle a generous pinch of ground turmeric over the cauliflower, along with a pinch of salt and a dash of freshly ground black pepper. Toss the ingredients gently to ensure even distribution of the spices.

Spread the seasoned cauliflower evenly on a baking sheet, allowing ample space between the florets to ensure proper roasting. Place the sheet in the preheated oven and let the magic unfold. As the cauliflower roasts, periodically check and gently toss the florets for even cooking. The roasting process typically takes around 20-25 minutes, depending on your desired level of crispiness.

Savoring the Culinary Delight:

Once the roasted turmeric cauliflower emerges from the oven, prepare to indulge your senses. The enticing aroma will beckon you, and the sight of the golden-hued florets will be a feast for the eyes. With a gentle crunch and a burst of flavors, each bite offers a harmonious medley of sweet, savory, and slightly peppery notes. Enjoy the roasted turmeric cauliflower as a side dish, a wholesome snack, or even as a topping for salads and grain bowls.

Roasted turmeric cauliflower is a testament to the magic that can be created when simple ingredients are thoughtfully combined and prepared. This delightful side or snack not only satisfies cravings but also nourishes the body with its healthful properties. Embark on a culinary journey with roasted turmeric cauliflower, and allow its captivating blend of flavors and textures to redefine your appreciation for this versatile vegetable.

Roasted Beet and Goat Cheese Salad

In the realm of culinary artistry, the combination of vibrant roasted beets and creamy goat cheese creates a symphony of flavors and textures that is nothing short of delightful. This captivating salad transcends ordinary dining, offering a sensory experience that marries earthy sweetness with tangy creaminess, making it a perfect side dish or a refreshing snack.

Elevating the Humble Beet:

Beets, often overlooked, are culinary gems that hold both aesthetic and nutritional value. Their rich, jewel-like colors and earthy flavors can be enhanced through roasting, a technique that intensifies their sweetness and transforms them into a tender delight. Packed with essential nutrients like fiber, vitamins, and antioxidants, beets contribute not only to the flavor profile but also to the healthfulness of the dish.

The Creamy Tang of Goat Cheese:

Goat cheese, with its tangy and velvety qualities, is the perfect companion to roasted beets. Its creamy texture provides a delightful contrast to the firmness of the beets, while its subtle tanginess adds depth to the overall flavor experience. The marriage of these two ingredients creates a harmonious blend that tickles the taste buds and leaves a lasting impression.

Crafting the Roasted Beet and Goat Cheese Salad:

Creating this exquisite salad is an endeavor that reaps both culinary and visual rewards. Begin by selecting fresh, firm beets of various colors, if available, to create a visually appealing palette. Preheat your oven to around 375°F (190°C). Scrub the beets clean and remove any rough patches, but leave the skin intact to preserve their color and nutrients.

Wrap each beet individually in aluminum foil and place them on a baking sheet. Roast in the preheated oven for approximately 45 to 60 minutes, or until a fork easily pierces through the beets. Once roasted, allow them to cool slightly before peeling and slicing them into rounds or wedges.

Arrange the roasted beet slices on a serving platter or individual plates, creating a captivating mosaic of colors. Next, crumble or thinly slice the goat cheese and scatter it generously over the beets, allowing the creaminess to mingle with the roasted goodness.

Dressing for Success:

To further enhance the flavors of the salad, a simple vinaigrette can be the perfect finishing touch. A balsamic vinegar-based dressing, with its tangy sweetness, complements the earthy tones of the beets and the goat cheese exquisitely. Drizzle the dressing over the salad, allowing it to infuse every bite with its vibrant flavor.

A Feast for the Senses:

With each forkful of roasted beet and goat cheese salad, you embark on a culinary journey that engages all your senses. The sight of the colorful beet slices, the creamy texture of the goat cheese, the tantalizing aroma, and the explosion of flavors in your mouth all contribute to a dining experience that is truly delightful.

The roasted beet and goat cheese salad stands as a testament to the art of culinary pairing and the magic that can be achieved through thoughtful ingredient selection and preparation. Whether enjoyed as a side dish at a gourmet dinner or as a refreshing snack on a warm day, this salad transcends mere sustenance to become a memorable gastronomic masterpiece.

Spiced Chickpea Popcorn

In the world of innovative culinary creations, spiced chickpea popcorn emerges as a captivating and irresistible treat that seamlessly blends healthfulness with indulgence. This delightful fusion takes the humble chickpea and transforms it into a crunchy, flavorful snack that is perfect for satisfying cravings and adding a unique twist to your snacking repertoire.

Chickpeas: A Nutritional Powerhouse:

Chickpeas, also known as garbanzo beans, are a nutritional powerhouse, packed with protein, fiber, vitamins, and minerals. Their mild, nutty flavor serves as a versatile canvas for culinary experimentation. By roasting them until crispy, chickpeas take on an entirely new dimension, becoming a crunchy and satisfying alternative to traditional popcorn.

The Art of Spicing:

The heart of spiced chickpea popcorn lies in the art of seasoning. Here, creativity knows no bounds. Whether you opt for a smoky paprika-infused blend, a fiery chili-lime medley, or an aromatic curry-spiced fusion, the key is to balance flavors and enhance the natural taste of the chickpeas. Spices not only tantalize the taste buds but also infuse the chickpeas with layers of complexity, transforming a simple legume into a gourmet snack.

Crafting Spiced Chickpea Popcorn:

Creating this delectable snack is a rewarding endeavor that requires minimal effort and yields maximum satisfaction. Begin by draining and rinsing a can of chickpeas. Pat them dry thoroughly using a kitchen towel or paper towels to ensure they roast to a crisp texture. Preheat your oven to around 400°F (200°C).

In a bowl, toss the chickpeas with a drizzle of olive oil to coat them evenly. This helps the spices adhere and promotes even roasting. Now, it's time to add your chosen spices. Whether you prefer a blend of cumin and coriander, a touch of garlic powder, or a smattering of nutritional yeast for a cheesy note, generously sprinkle the seasoning over the chickpeas and toss to distribute.

Spread the seasoned chickpeas on a baking sheet lined with parchment paper in a single layer. This allows each chickpea to roast evenly and achieve that desired crunch. Roast the chickpeas in the preheated oven for approximately 25-30 minutes, stirring occasionally to prevent burning.

The Sensory Experience:

As the spiced chickpea popcorn roasts, your kitchen will be enveloped in a tantalizing aroma that signals the impending delight. Once out of the oven, allow the chickpeas to cool slightly before diving in. The result is a medley of textures and flavors—crispy on the outside, tender on the inside, and bursting with the excitement of the spices.

Spiced chickpea popcorn stands as a testament to the culinary magic that can be achieved through creative pairing and skillful seasoning. This delightful snack not only satisfies your cravings but also offers a nutritious alternative to traditional snacks. As you explore the endless possibilities of spice combinations, you embark on a flavorful journey that elevates the humble chickpea to a coveted treat. Whether enjoyed during movie nights, gatherings, or as a midday pick-me-up, spiced chickpea popcorn promises a symphony of flavors that will leave you craving more.

Chapter 6: Meal Plans and Weekly Menus

In the fast-paced modern world, where time is a precious commodity and health is a priority, meal planning and creating weekly menus have emerged as essential tools for individuals and families seeking to maintain a balanced and nourishing diet. These practices offer not only convenience and organization but also the opportunity to make informed food choices and cultivate a healthier relationship with food.

The Art of Meal Planning

Meal planning is the strategic approach of mapping out what you'll eat over a designated period, often a week. It involves taking into account your dietary preferences, nutritional needs, and the ingredients you have on hand. By investing a little time upfront, you can save yourself from the stress of last-minute meal decisions and impulsive, less health-conscious choices.

1. Efficiency: Meal planning streamlines your grocery shopping by creating a precise list of ingredients you'll need. This not only saves time but also reduces food waste since you're purchasing only what you intend to use.

2. Nutritional Balance: Crafting well-rounded meal plans allows you to ensure you're getting a variety of nutrients from different food groups. Balancing proteins, carbohydrates, healthy fats, and a rainbow of fruits and vegetables becomes more manageable.

3. Portion Control: Meal planning encourages mindful portioning, helping you avoid overeating and promoting weight management.

Weekly Menus: Your Culinary Blueprint**

A weekly menu is like a roadmap for your culinary journey throughout the week. It breaks down your meal plan into daily specifics, offering a clear guide for what you'll be eating and when. Weekly menus provide structure and consistency to your eating habits, making it easier to stay on track with your health and dietary goals.

1. Diverse Choices: A well-designed weekly menu ensures you're not stuck in a culinary rut. You can incorporate a range of flavors, cuisines, and ingredients to keep your meals exciting and enjoyable.

2. Time Management: With a weekly menu, you can allocate time for meal preparation, making cooking a less daunting task even on busy days.

3. Special Occasions and Goals: Weekly menus can be tailored to accommodate special occasions, dietary restrictions, or specific health objectives, such as weight loss, muscle gain, or heart-healthy eating.

Creating Your Meal Planning Routine

Getting started with meal planning and weekly menus may seem overwhelming, but with a systematic approach, it becomes an empowering habit.

1. Assess Your Needs: Consider your dietary goals, preferences, and the number of meals you need to plan for each day.

2. Select Recipes: Choose recipes that align with your objectives and suit your cooking skills. Online resources, cookbooks, and food apps offer a plethora of ideas.

3. Compile Ingredients: Create a comprehensive shopping list based on the recipes you've selected, ensuring you have all the necessary ingredients.

4. Preparation: Dedicate a specific time for meal prep, whether it's on weekends or a designated evening during the week. Chop vegetables, marinate proteins, and cook staples in advance to streamline cooking throughout the week.

5. Flexibility: While planning is essential, allow for flexibility. Life can be unpredictable, so be prepared to adjust your plans when necessary.

In a world filled with numerous demands on our time, meal plans and weekly menus provide a sense of control over our nutrition and well-being. They empower us to make intentional food choices, cultivate culinary creativity, and foster a healthier relationship with what we eat. Whether you're a seasoned chef or a novice cook, embracing these practices can lead to a more efficient, satisfying, and nourishing way of eating.

One–Week Low FODMAP Vegetarian Meal Plan

The low FODMAP diet has gained recognition for its ability to provide relief to individuals dealing with irritable bowel syndrome (IBS) and digestive sensitivities. FODMAPs, which stands for Fermentable Oligosaccharides, Disaccharides, Monosaccharides, and Polyols, are certain types of carbohydrates that can trigger digestive discomfort in some people. Adopting a low FODMAP diet can be especially challenging for vegetarians, but with thoughtful planning and creative choices, it's entirely possible to enjoy a week of delicious, gut-friendly vegetarian meals.

Understanding the Low FODMAP Diet

The low FODMAP diet involves avoiding foods high in specific types of carbohydrates that are known to ferment in the gut and potentially lead to symptoms like bloating, gas, and abdominal pain. While many fruits, vegetables, grains, and legumes are off-limits, there is a wide range of options that are naturally low in FODMAPs and can be enjoyed in a vegetarian meal plan.

A One-Week Low FODMAP Vegetarian Meal Plan

Day 1: Breakfast
- Scrambled eggs with spinach and cherry tomatoes

- Gluten-free toast
- Green tea

Lunch
- Quinoa salad with grilled zucchini, carrots, and a lemon vinaigrette
- Mixed greens with cucumber and olive oil

Dinner
- Roasted tofu with green beans and mashed potatoes (using lactose-free butter)
- Orange slices for dessert

Day 2: Breakfast
- Greek yogurt (lactose-free) with blueberries and a sprinkle of chia seeds
- Gluten-free oatmeal

Lunch
- Spinach and arugula salad with roasted butternut squash, walnuts, and a balsamic vinaigrette

Dinner

- Stuffed bell peppers with rice, firm tofu, and zucchini
- Sliced strawberries

Day 3: Breakfast

- Smoothie with lactose-free yogurt, banana, strawberries, and a small handful of almonds

Lunch

- Low FODMAP vegetable soup (using garlic-infused oil)
- Gluten-free crackers

Dinner

- Grilled eggplant and zucchini skewers with a side of quinoa
- Pineapple chunks

Day 4: Breakfast

- Peanut butter (watch portion size) on gluten-free toast
- Kiwi slices

Lunch

- Mixed greens with sliced oranges, walnuts, and a citrus vinaigrette
- Grilled tofu

Dinner

- Baked potato with lactose-free sour cream and a side salad

Day 5: Breakfast

- Smoothie with lactose-free yogurt, pineapple, and spinach
- Rice cakes

Lunch

- Stir-fried rice with carrots, bell peppers, and scallions (use only the green parts)
- Almond-crusted tofu

Dinner

- Low FODMAP vegetable and lentil curry
- Steamed basmati rice

Day 6: Breakfast

- Chia seed pudding made with lactose-free milk, topped with raspberries
- Gluten-free granola

Lunch

- Tomato and mozzarella salad with fresh basil (moderate portion of mozzarella)
- Quinoa and cucumber salad

Dinner

- Grilled portobello mushrooms with polenta and sautéed spinach

Day 7: Breakfast

- Rice cakes with almond butter and sliced strawberries
- Herbal tea

Lunch

- Spinach and mixed greens with grilled eggplant, cherry tomatoes, and a lemon-tahini dressing

Dinner

- Zucchini noodles with homemade low FODMAP pesto (omit garlic, use garlic-infused oil)
- Mixed berries for dessert

Important Considerations

When following a low FODMAP diet, it's crucial to work with a healthcare professional or registered dietitian to ensure you're meeting your nutritional needs and avoiding potential triggers. Additionally, portion sizes and individual tolerances may vary, so it's essential to listen to your body and make adjustments as needed.

As you embark on this one-week low FODMAP vegetarian meal plan, you're not only nurturing your gut health but also indulging in a variety of flavorful, wholesome, and satisfying dishes. With creativity and careful planning, you can enjoy a week of delicious and gut-friendly vegetarian eating that supports your well-being.

Two-Week Digestive Reset Menu

Taking a mindful approach to your diet by focusing on gut health and digestive wellness can have a transformative impact on your overall well-being. In this two-week digestive reset menu, we'll explore nourishing and easily digestible meals enhanced by a variety of sauces, dressings, and condiments that not only elevate flavors but also support your digestive system.

Week 1

Day 1:

- Breakfast: Overnight oats with almond milk, chia seeds, and sliced bananas.
- Lunch: Spinach salad with grilled chicken, cucumber, and a light lemon vinaigrette.
- Dinner: Baked salmon with roasted sweet potatoes and steamed asparagus.

Day 2:

- Breakfast: Smoothie with spinach, pineapple, ginger, and coconut water.
- Lunch: Quinoa and vegetable stir-fry with tofu and a tamari glaze.
- Dinner: Grilled turkey burgers with a side of mixed greens and a balsamic reduction.

Day 3:

- Breakfast: Greek yogurt with raspberries, walnuts, and a drizzle of honey.
- Lunch: Lentil soup with a side of gluten-free crackers.
- Dinner: Zucchini noodles with sautéed shrimp and a homemade pesto (garlic-free).

Day 4:

- Breakfast: Scrambled eggs with sautéed spinach and a slice of gluten-free toast.
- Lunch: Brown rice bowl with black beans, avocado, and a tahini drizzle.
- Dinner: Grilled chicken with quinoa pilaf and steamed broccoli.

Day 5:

- Breakfast: Smoothie with banana, blueberries, almond milk, and a spoonful of almond butter.
- Lunch: Mixed greens with grilled vegetables, chickpeas, and a lemon-turmeric dressing.
- Dinner: Baked cod with roasted Brussels sprouts and a squeeze of fresh lemon.

Week 2

Day 6:
- Breakfast: Chia seed pudding with lactose-free yogurt and mixed berries.
- Lunch: Spinach and arugula salad with grilled portobello mushrooms and a balsamic glaze.
- Dinner: Stir-fried tofu and vegetables in a ginger soy sauce served over brown rice.

Day 7:
- Breakfast: Rice cakes with avocado slices and a sprinkle of sesame seeds.
- Lunch: Tomato and mozzarella salad with basil and a drizzle of olive oil.
- Dinner: Lemon herb grilled shrimp with quinoa and steamed green beans.

Day 8:

- Breakfast: Omelette with sautéed bell peppers, spinach, and feta cheese.

- Lunch: Butternut squash soup with a side of gluten-free bread.

- Dinner: Grilled tempeh with a kale and almond salad, dressed with a light citrus vinaigrette.

Day 9:

- Breakfast: Smoothie with mixed berries, spinach, and coconut water.

- Lunch: Brown rice bowl with roasted vegetables, hummus, and a sprinkle of pumpkin seeds.

- Dinner: Herb-marinated grilled chicken with a side of mashed cauliflower.

Day 10:

- Breakfast: Quinoa porridge with almond milk, sliced almonds, and diced peaches.

- Lunch: Mixed greens with grilled chicken, cherry tomatoes, and a lemon-tahini dressing.

- Dinner: Seared salmon with quinoa and sautéed spinach.

Important Note:

During this two-week digestive reset, be mindful of your individual dietary needs and sensitivities. Consult with a healthcare professional or registered dietitian before making significant changes to your diet, especially if you have any underlying health conditions. The goal of this menu is to emphasize whole, nutrient-rich foods and digestive-friendly ingredients while exploring a variety of sauces, dressings, and condiments to enhance your meals and support your digestive well-being.

Customizable Meal Planning Template

Meal planning is the cornerstone of efficient and intentional eating, helping you save time, reduce stress, and make healthier food choices. Crafting a customizable meal planning template is like designing your personal culinary roadmap, guiding you through a week of nourishing meals and satisfying flavors. Whether you're a busy professional, a dedicated parent, or simply looking to optimize your eating habits, a well-designed meal planning template can be your secret weapon for success.

Step 1: Setting the Stage

Before diving into the template, consider your unique needs, preferences, and dietary goals. Are you looking to focus on weight management, muscle gain, or digestive health? Are there specific foods you need to avoid due to allergies or sensitivities? Understanding your objectives will help you tailor your meal plan accordingly.

Step 2: The Framework

Create a basic structure for your meal plan template. This could be a table divided into days of the week, with columns for breakfast, lunch, dinner, and snacks. Leave additional space for notes, ingredients, or special instructions.

Step 3: Personalize Your Plan

Now it's time to fill in the details. Here's a breakdown of each section:

Breakfast:
- Choose a balance of protein, healthy fats, and complex carbohydrates. Examples: smoothies, yogurt bowls, eggs, oatmeal.

Lunch:
- Incorporate lean proteins, whole grains, and a variety of colorful vegetables. Examples: salads, wraps, grain bowls, soups.

Dinner:
- Focus on well-rounded meals with lean proteins, complex carbs, and plenty of veggies. Examples: grilled chicken with quinoa and roasted vegetables, stir-fry, baked fish with sweet potato.

Snacks:

- Opt for nutrient-dense snacks that keep you satisfied between meals. Examples: nuts, fruits, veggie sticks with hummus, Greek yogurt.

Step 4: Embrace Flexibility

Your meal planning template should be a guide, not a rigid set of rules. Allow room for flexibility and spontaneity. If you're trying a new recipe or dining out, simply adjust your plan accordingly.

Step 5: Flavorful Enhancements

Here's where sauces, dressings, and condiments come into play. Dedicate a section of your template to highlight the flavor-boosting elements of each meal:

- **Sauces and Dressings:** List the sauces or dressings you'll use to elevate your meals. Examples: balsamic vinaigrette, tahini drizzle, salsa.

- **Condiments:** Include any condiments or toppings that add a delightful twist. Examples: sliced avocado, chopped nuts, grated Parmesan.

Step 6: Grocery List Integration

To streamline your shopping, create a space on your template for a grocery list. As you plan your meals, jot down the ingredients you'll need for each recipe. This will help you stay organized and prevent over-purchasing.

Step 7: Theme Nights or Cuisine Exploration

Consider incorporating theme nights or exploring different cuisines throughout the week. Mexican Monday, Thai Tuesday, or Meatless Wednesday can infuse variety and excitement into your meal plan.

Step 8: Reflection and Adaptation

At the end of each week, reflect on your meal plan. What worked well? What could be improved? Use this feedback to refine your template for the following week.

Your meal planning template is a tool designed to make your life easier and your meals more enjoyable. As you embrace the art of meal planning, you'll find that having a customizable template at your fingertips empowers you to savor delicious, balanced, and satisfying meals while maintaining a sense of organization and control in your culinary journey.

Chapter 7: Navigating Dining Out and Social Situations

Dining out and engaging in social situations often involve a blend of etiquette, communication skills, and cultural awareness. Whether you're meeting friends, colleagues, or new acquaintances, mastering the art of navigating these scenarios can enhance your overall experience and leave a positive impression on others. Here are some tips to help you navigate dining out and social situations with confidence:

1. Planning Ahead:
  - Research the restaurant or venue beforehand to get an idea of the menu, atmosphere, and dress code.
  - Consider any dietary restrictions or preferences you or your companions may have, and check if the restaurant can accommodate them.

2. Making Reservations:

- If the occasion calls for it, make reservations in advance to ensure you have a table, especially at popular establishments.

- Communicate any special requirements or preferences when making the reservation, such as seating preferences or occasions being celebrated.

3. Arrival and Greetings:

- Arrive on time or a few minutes early to show respect for others' schedules.

- Greet your companions warmly, using appropriate handshakes or gestures based on cultural norms.

4. Seating Etiquette:

- Wait for the host or hostess to indicate where you should sit, especially in formal settings.

- Allow elders, guests of honor, or those with special needs to choose their seats first.

5. Ordering Food:

- If you're the host or if it's your idea to dine out, take the lead in suggesting dishes or sharing recommendations from the menu.

- Be mindful of others' preferences and dietary restrictions when suggesting shared dishes.

6. Table Manners:

- Use utensils properly, starting from the outside and working your way in for each course.

- Chew with your mouth closed, and avoid talking with food in your mouth.

- Take cues from others on the pace of eating, so you don't finish your meal much earlier or later than everyone else.

7. Engaging in Conversation:

- Practice active listening and engage in meaningful conversations with those around you.

- Avoid controversial or sensitive topics unless you know the group well and are certain they're appropriate.

8. Technology Use:

- Keep your phone on silent or vibrate and avoid checking it frequently during the meal.

- Be present in the moment and focus on enjoying the company of your companions.

9. Paying the Bill:

- If you initiated the gathering, be prepared to pay the bill unless someone else offers.

- If splitting the bill, suggest a fair and organized way to divide the expenses.

10. Expressing Gratitude:

- Thank your companions for their company and the experience at the end of the meal.

- A simple thank you note or text message after the gathering can leave a positive lasting impression.

11. Cultural Sensitivity:

- Be aware of cultural norms and customs, especially if dining with individuals from diverse backgrounds.

- Avoid behaviors that might be considered disrespectful or offensive in certain cultures.

The key to successfully navigating dining out and social situations lies in respect, consideration, and adaptability. By following these guidelines and being attentive to the comfort of others, you can create enjoyable and memorable experiences for everyone involved.

Tips for Eating Low FODMAP at Restaurants

Eating out can be a delightful experience, but it can pose challenges for individuals following a low FODMAP diet. FODMAPs (Fermentable Oligosaccharides, Disaccharides, Monosaccharides, and Polyols) are a group of short-chain carbohydrates that can trigger digestive symptoms in some people, especially those with irritable bowel syndrome (IBS). If you're on a low FODMAP diet, here are some valuable tips to help you enjoy dining out and social gatherings while managing your dietary needs:

1. Research Restaurants:

- Before choosing a restaurant, research their menu online or call ahead to inquire about low FODMAP options. Many establishments are becoming more accommodating to dietary restrictions.

2. Communication is Key:

- Inform your server about your dietary requirements. Politely explain that you're on a low FODMAP diet and ask if they can help you identify suitable menu choices.

3. Customize Your Order:

- Don't hesitate to ask for modifications to dishes to make them low FODMAP. For example, request no onions, garlic, or high FODMAP sauces.

4. Choose Wisely:

- Opt for dishes that are naturally low in FODMAPs, such as grilled meats, fish, seafood, and most vegetables (e.g., carrots, spinach, zucchini).

- Be cautious with dishes that may contain hidden sources of FODMAPs, like soups, gravies, and dressings.

5. Avoid Hidden FODMAPs:

- Educate yourself about common high FODMAP ingredients and hidden sources, like certain additives and sweeteners.

- Stay vigilant when choosing condiments, marinades, and sides.

6. Beverage Choices:

- Stick to low FODMAP beverages like water, tea, or coffee without high FODMAP additives.

- Be cautious with alcoholic drinks, as some mixers and additives can contain FODMAPs.

7. Portion Control:

- Pay attention to portion sizes, as consuming large quantities of even low FODMAP foods can trigger symptoms.

- Consider sharing larger dishes with others or opting for smaller portions.

8. Ask Questions:

- Don't hesitate to ask your server questions about ingredients, preparation methods, and potential FODMAP content of dishes.

- A well-informed server can help ensure a safer dining experience.

9. Savor the Sides:

- Choose simple side dishes like steamed vegetables, baked potatoes, or plain rice to complement your meal.

10. Be Prepared:

- If you're unsure about the options available, consider eating a small low FODMAP snack before you go out to ensure you're not too hungry when making choices.

11. Express Appreciation:

- Thank the staff for their assistance and understanding in accommodating your dietary needs. Positive interactions can lead to better experiences in the future.

12. Bring a Dining Card:

- Consider carrying a card that explains your dietary needs in detail. This can be especially helpful when dining in restaurants where language barriers may exist.

Dining out on a low FODMAP diet is entirely possible with careful planning, effective communication, and a willingness to explore various options. By advocating for your needs and making informed choices, you can savor delicious meals while prioritizing your health and well-being in social situations.

Communicating Dietary Needs with Others

Communicating your dietary needs effectively is essential for ensuring a pleasant dining experience while maintaining your health and well-being. Whether you're managing food allergies, intolerances, preferences, or following a specific diet, clear communication can help you and those around you make informed choices. Here are some strategies for effectively communicating your dietary needs in various social settings:

1. Plan Ahead:

- If you know you'll be dining out or attending a social event, plan in advance. Research the restaurant's menu or ask the host about the planned food options to assess their compatibility with your dietary requirements.

2. Be Direct and Clear:

- When discussing your dietary needs, be concise and straightforward. Use clear language and avoid excessive details that may confuse others.

3. Choose the Right Time:

- If you have complex dietary needs, choose a suitable time to discuss them with your host or the restaurant staff. Arriving early or calling ahead can provide ample time for a thorough conversation.

4. Politeness and Respect:

- Approach the conversation with a positive and respectful tone. Express your gratitude for their consideration and willingness to accommodate your dietary needs.

5. Ask Questions:

- Don't hesitate to ask questions about ingredients, preparation methods, and possible substitutions. Understanding the menu better can help you make informed decisions.

6. Use Allergy Cards or Apps:

- If you have severe allergies or dietary restrictions, consider using allergy cards or mobile apps that explain your needs in a concise and easily understandable manner.

7. Offer Solutions:

- Propose alternatives or modifications that could make a dish suitable for your dietary needs. This can make it easier for the kitchen staff to accommodate your request.

8. Educate About Your Needs:

- Share relevant information about your dietary needs, especially if they're less common. This helps others understand the reasons behind your choices.

9. Dine with Empathetic Companions:

- When dining with friends or colleagues, choose people who are understanding and supportive of your dietary needs. This can create a more comfortable and inclusive atmosphere.

10. Thank Your Host or Server:

- Express gratitude to your host or server for their efforts in accommodating your dietary requirements. A simple "thank you" goes a long way in fostering positive interactions.

11. Stay Open-Minded:

- While it's important to communicate your needs, be flexible and open to options that may not be an exact match. Sometimes, creative solutions can lead to delightful dining experiences.

12. Confidence and Assertiveness:

- Approach the conversation with confidence, and don't be afraid to assert your needs. Remember that your health and well-being are top priorities.

13. Lead by Example:

- Share your dietary needs and preferences with others in a non-judgmental way. By leading by example, you can help create a culture of understanding and respect around food choices.

14. Express Gratitude:

- After the meal or event, take a moment to thank your host, server, or chef for their accommodations. Positive feedback encourages them to continue being mindful of dietary needs.

Effective communication about your dietary needs allows you to enjoy dining out and socializing without compromising your health. By following these strategies, you can foster understanding, cooperation, and a more inclusive dining experience for yourself and those around you.

Low FODMAP Party and Gathering Ideas

Hosting or attending a social gathering while following a low FODMAP diet doesn't mean you have to miss out on delicious food and enjoyable experiences. With some creativity and thoughtful planning, you can create a memorable and inclusive event that caters to everyone's dietary needs. Here are some low FODMAP party and gathering ideas to help you navigate social situations with ease:

1. Menu Planning:

- Research low FODMAP foods and ingredients to create a diverse and flavorful menu.

- Incorporate naturally low FODMAP options such as grilled meats, seafood, poultry, vegetables (e.g., carrots, bell peppers), fruits (e.g., strawberries, grapes), and lactose-free dairy products.

2. Appetizers and Snacks:

- Offer a variety of gluten-free and low FODMAP appetizers like cheese platters, olives, nuts, and vegetable sticks with dip.

- Create a colorful fruit platter with low FODMAP fruits like pineapple, kiwi, and berries.

3. Beverages:

- Provide a selection of low FODMAP drinks such as water, herbal teas, and fruit-infused water.

- Consider making mocktails using fresh fruit juices and soda water.

4. Main Course:

- Grill or roast meats, fish, or poultry with flavorful low FODMAP marinades or rubs.

- Offer a build-your-own taco or burrito station with corn tortillas, grilled meat, lettuce, tomatoes, and lactose-free cheese.

5. Sides:

- Serve roasted or steamed vegetables like carrots, green beans, and zucchini.

- Prepare a quinoa or rice salad with low FODMAP vegetables, herbs, and a lemon vinaigrette.

6. Desserts:

- Create a dessert bar with low FODMAP options like dark chocolate, rice cakes, and fruit skewers.

- Bake gluten-free and low FODMAP desserts using almond flour or gluten-free oats.

7. Allergy-Friendly Labels:

- Label each dish with its ingredients to help guests identify safe options.

- Clearly mark any dishes that may contain common allergens or high FODMAP ingredients.

8. Communication:

- Inform your guests in advance about the low FODMAP theme and ask if anyone has specific dietary needs or allergies.

- Share information about the low FODMAP diet and its benefits to help guests understand its significance.

9. Interactive Cooking Stations:

- Set up a DIY pizza-making station with gluten-free crusts and low FODMAP toppings.

- Create a "make your own salad" station with a variety of low FODMAP ingredients and dressings.

10. Themed Gatherings:

- Host a backyard BBQ featuring grilled low FODMAP meats, vegetable skewers, and potato salad made with lactose-free mayo.

- Organize a picnic with an assortment of fresh fruits, gluten-free sandwiches, and snacks.

11. Outdoor Picnics:

- Pack portable low FODMAP foods such as rice crackers, cheese, grapes, and sliced turkey for a hassle-free outdoor gathering.

12. Catering Assistance:

- If hosting feels overwhelming, consider working with a catering service that specializes in dietary restrictions to ensure a seamless and delicious experience.

13. Engage in Activities:

- Plan engaging activities like board games, karaoke, or outdoor games to ensure that the focus isn't solely on food.

14. Collect Feedback:

- After the gathering, ask for feedback from your guests to learn what worked well and how you can improve future low FODMAP events.

Hosting a low FODMAP party or gathering is a chance to showcase your culinary creativity while also promoting inclusivity for everyone's dietary needs. By putting thought into your menu and creating an enjoyable atmosphere, you can ensure a successful and memorable event for all your guests.

Conclusion

In conclusion, the creation of the Low FODMAP Vegetarian Cookbook represents a significant step forward in the realm of dietary inclusivity and culinary innovation. By combining the principles of the low FODMAP diet with the diverse and vibrant world of vegetarian cuisine, this cookbook has successfully addressed the dietary needs and preferences of a wide range of individuals, ultimately promoting better digestive health and overall well-being.

Through the thoughtful selection of ingredients and meticulous recipe development, the cookbook has demonstrated that a low FODMAP diet does not have to be restrictive or devoid of flavor. Instead, it showcases how creative culinary techniques can be harnessed to create delicious and satisfying meals that cater to individuals with sensitive digestive systems.

Furthermore, the Low FODMAP Vegetarian Cookbook has opened up new avenues for exploring the intersection of dietary requirements and ethical choices. By offering a variety of plant-based recipes that are both low in FODMAPs and rich in nutrients, it encourages individuals to make sustainable and health-conscious food choices while respecting their unique dietary needs.

As society continues to recognize the importance of personalized nutrition and the impact of diet on overall health, cookbooks like this one play a crucial role in providing practical guidance and inspiration. This cookbook serves as a valuable resource not only for those actively following a low FODMAP vegetarian diet, but also for healthcare professionals, dietitians, and chefs who seek to expand their culinary repertoire and offer inclusive options to their clients and customers.

In essence, the Low FODMAP Vegetarian Cookbook embodies the harmonious fusion of dietary science and gastronomic artistry. Its pages are a testament to the power of innovation and adaptation, demonstrating that the convergence of dietary restrictions and culinary exploration can lead to a healthier, more diverse, and more delicious way of eating. Whether one's motivations are rooted in health, ethics, or a combination of both, this cookbook stands as a testament to the fact that nourishing the body and delighting the palate can coexist in perfect harmony.

www.ingramcontent.com/pod-product-compliance
Lightning Source LLC
Chambersburg PA
CBHW070951250726
48663CB00002B/180